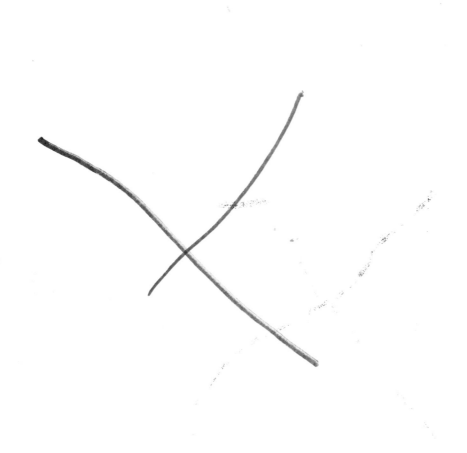

A Day in the Life of a...

Hairdresser

Carol Watson

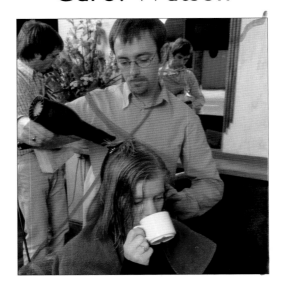

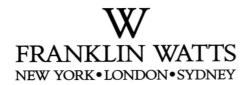

FRANKLIN WATTS

NEW YORK • LONDON • SYDNEY

This is Cascade Hair Salon.
It belongs to Paul.
He is a hairdresser and
works here with his team.

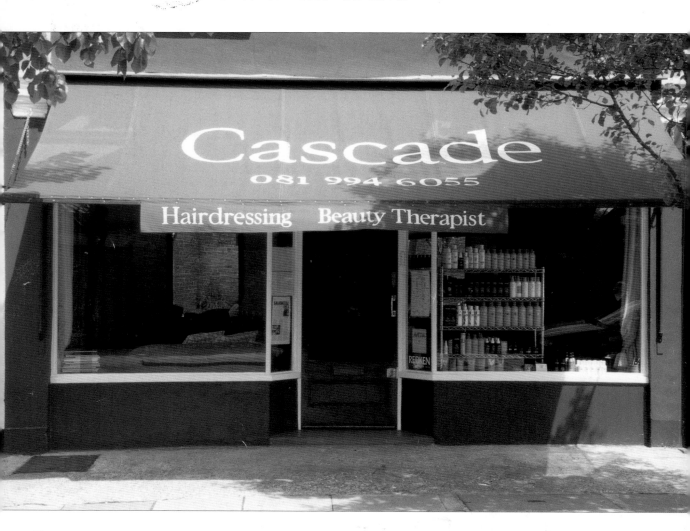

It's 8.00 a.m.
on Monday.
Paul starts the week
by talking to Michael,
one of the stylists,
about their clients.

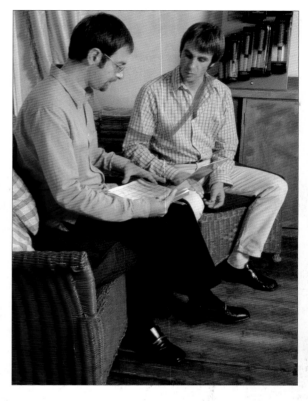

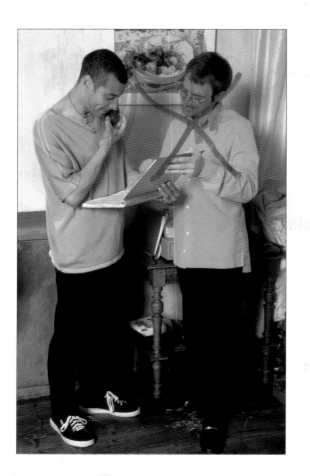

Next Paul looks
at the day's
appointments with
Patrick, a trainee.
"Who is booked
in for today?"
asks Paul.

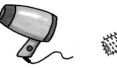

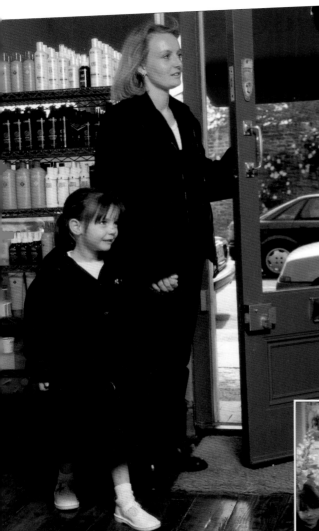

Paul's first client is Hannah. "I'm going to be a bridesmaid, today!" she tells Paul. "Then we'll make you look very special," he says.

Paul suggests some different hairstyles to Hannah.

4

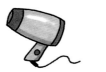

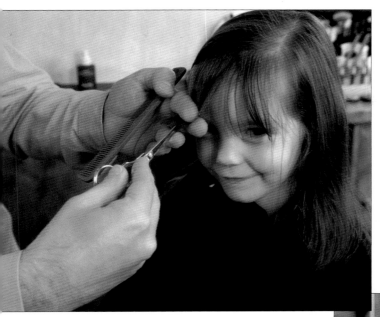

Once Hannah's
hair has been
washed, Paul
cuts it. Then he
gently gathers
her hair
into a bun.

Finally Hannah
is ready to go.
I'll put on some
spray," says Paul.
"That will keep
your hairstyle
in place."

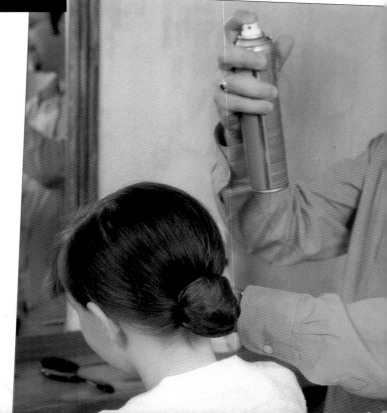

Meanwhile Michael is cutting Craig's hair.
"Do you want your hair
the same way as usual?" Michael asks.

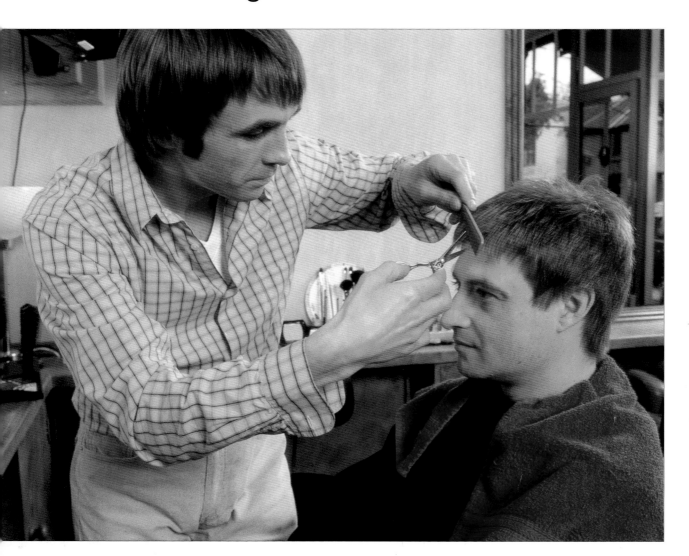

Another stylist, Kate, is working on Samantha's hair. She is putting colour into it to make the hair look lighter.

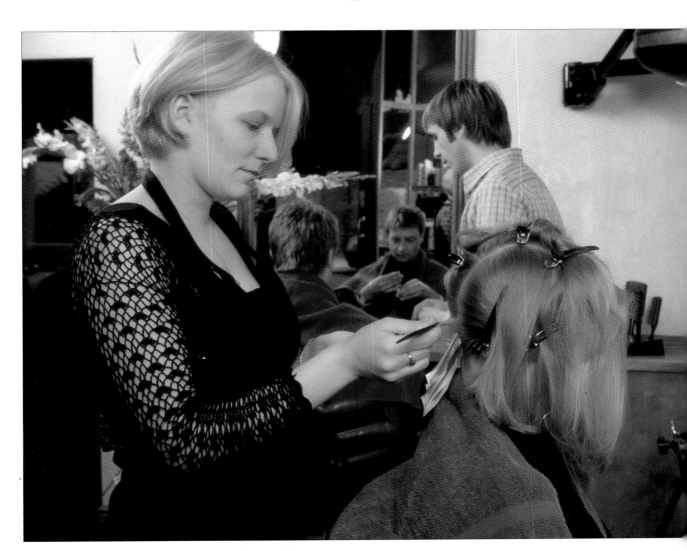

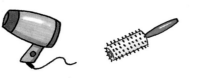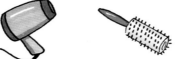

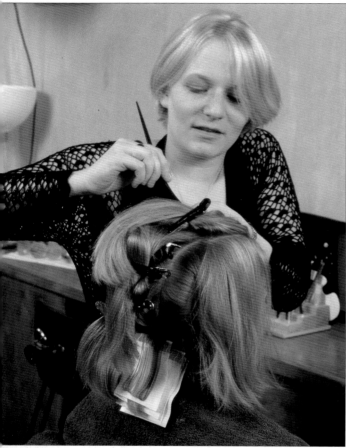

First Kate brushes the colour onto strips of Samantha's hair. Then she wraps each strip of hair in foils.

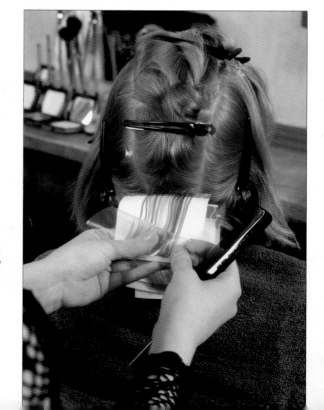

"Would you like a coffee?" Kate asks. "The colour highlights will take some time to work."

While they wait Kate and Paul have a quick snack in the garden.
"Samantha's hair will be ready in another twenty minutes," Kate tells Paul.

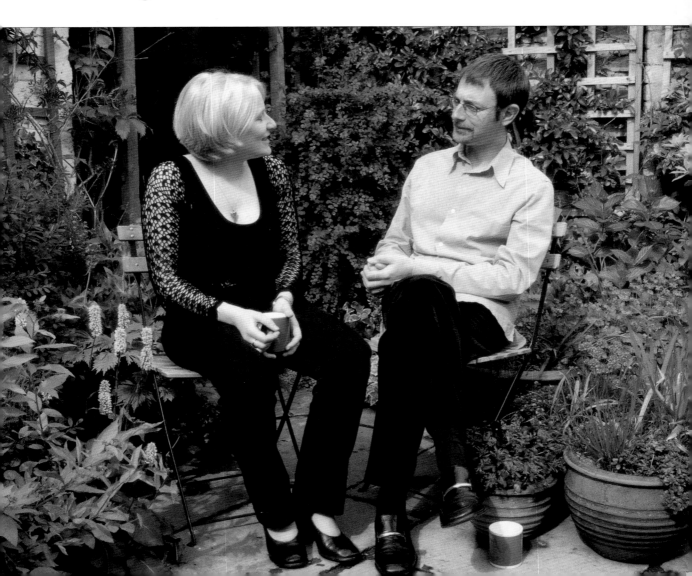

When the highlights are ready, Paul asks Patrick to wash Samantha's hair. Then Paul brushes and dries it into shape.

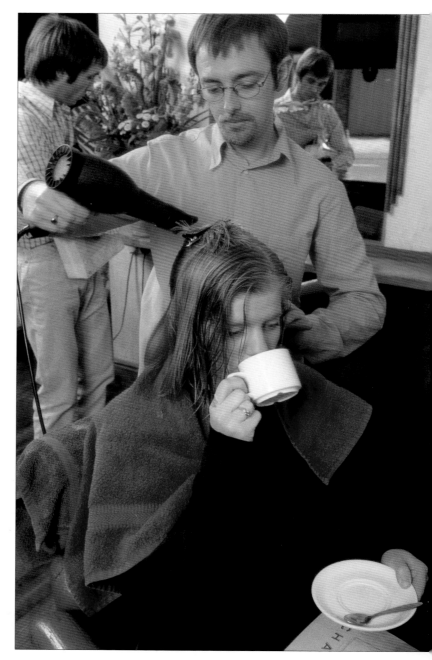

"That's it,"
says Paul.
"I've finished!"
He shows
Samantha her
hair at the
back by holding
up a mirror.
"That's lovely,"
 she says.
"Thank you."

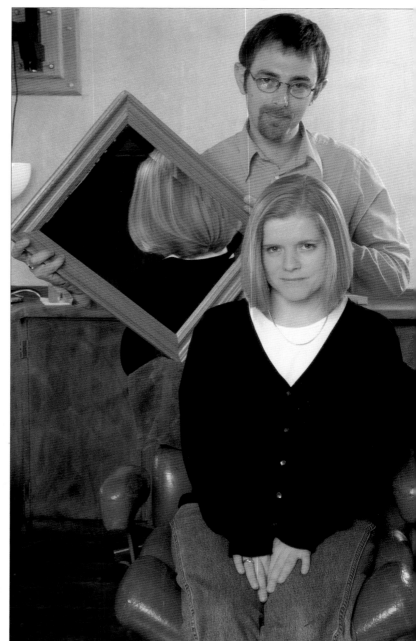

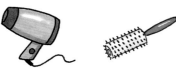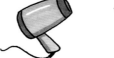

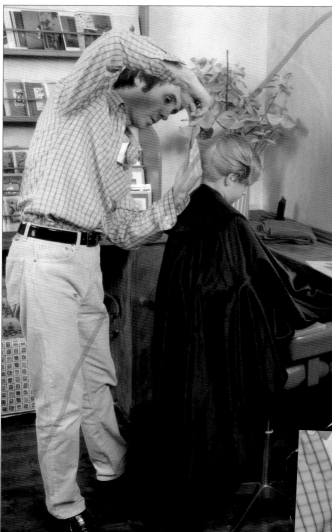

Matthew has
arrived for a trim.
When Michael has
finished the cut,
he brushes
Matthew's neck.

"That will make
sure you have
no ticklish hairs
down your
back!" he says.

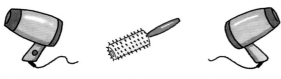

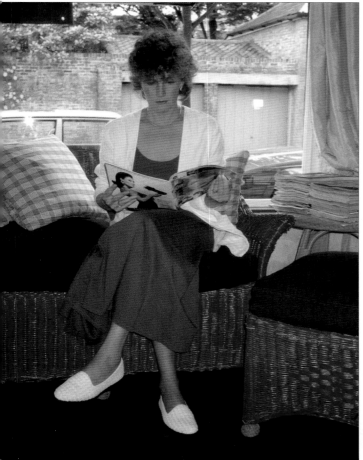

Paul's next client is Annabel. She is waiting in the reception area.

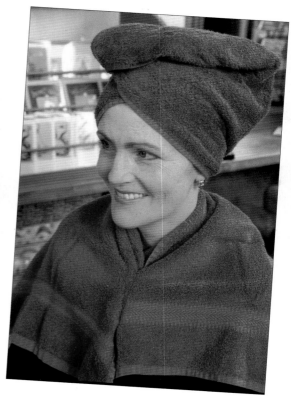

When Paul is ready for Annabel, Patrick washes her hair.

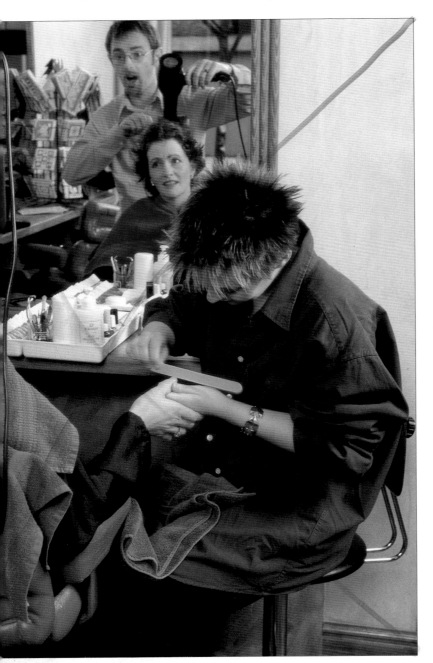

Then Paul
dries and styles
Annabel's hair
while Bonnie
manicures her
nails. Paul and
Annabel talk
about their
holidays.

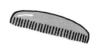

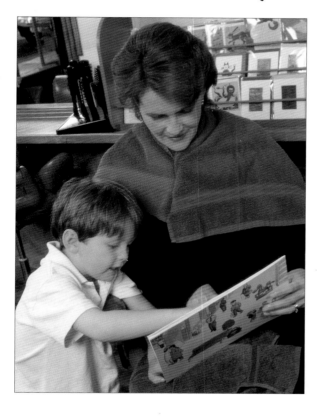

Annabel's children have arrived from school. "Hello Mum," says Charlie.

Annabel reads to her son while Asma washes Emily's hair.

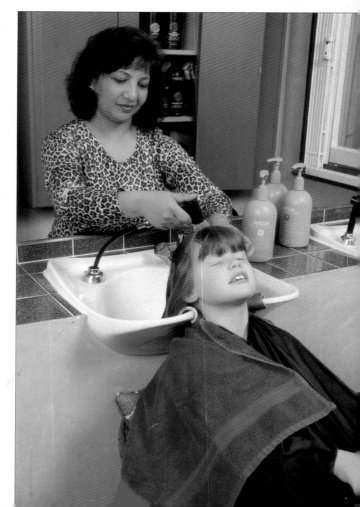

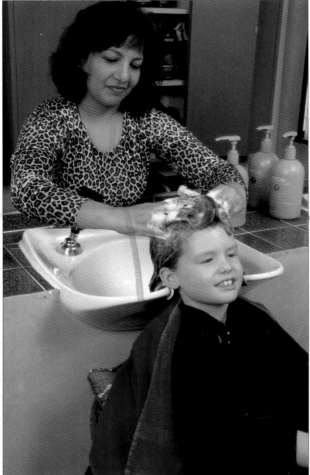

Asma spreads shampoo all over Emily's head and rubs the scalp with the tips of her fingers.

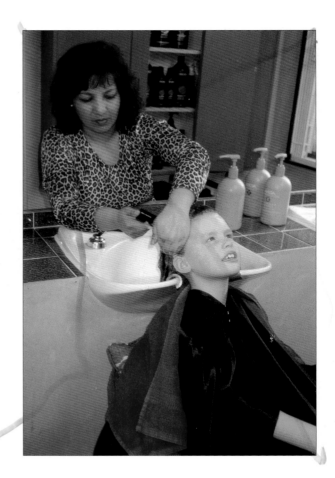

Then Asma rinses the hair well so that there is no trace of shampoo left.

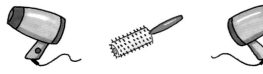

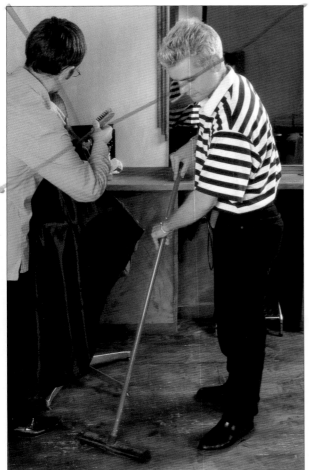

When Emily is ready Paul trims her hair. Russell, one of the juniors, sweeps the hair off the floor and tidies the salon.

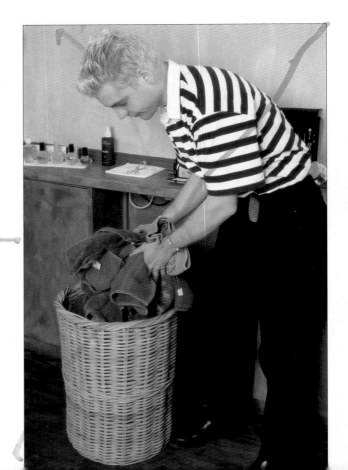

Now Annabel and her family
are ready to leave. "How much
do I owe you?" Annabel asks.
She pays the bill.

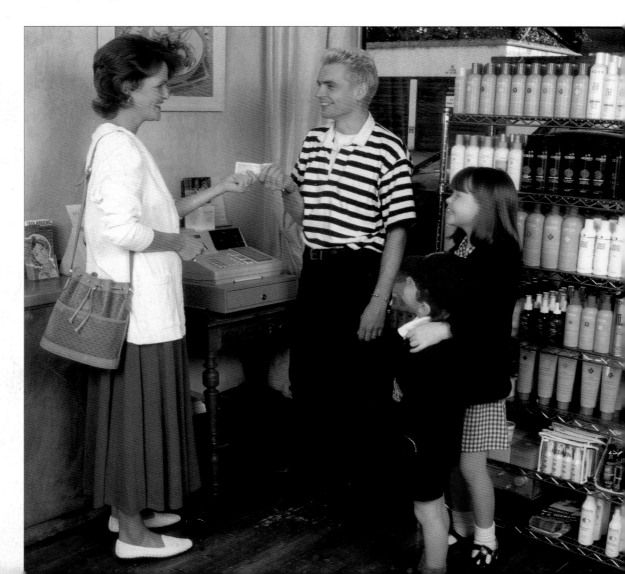

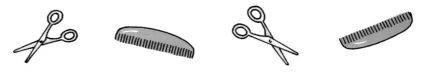

It's the end of the day and all the clients have gone. Paul puts up the blind on his hairdressing salon. "Time for home," he says.

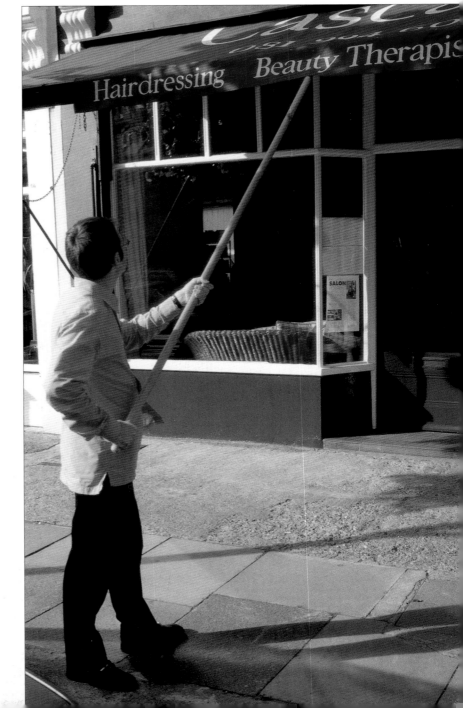

How to wash your hair like a hairdresser

Do you wash your own hair? Are you doing it properly? This is the way a hairdresser washes your hair. If you want your hair to look its best, this is the way to do it:

1. Wet your hair with warm water.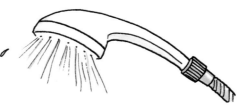

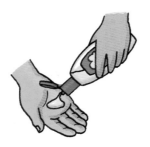 **2.** Pour about a teaspoonful of shampoo into one hand and spread it across both of your hands.

3. Dab the shampoo onto different parts of your head. Use a little water to make a "lather" and gently rub it over your head.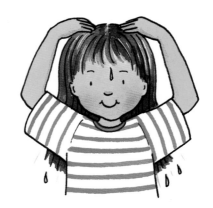

4. Rub the tips of your fingers in circular movements around your scalp.

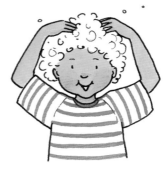

5. Next rinse your hair with clean water. Move your fingers through your hair as the water trickles through. Make sure you rinse out all the shampoo.

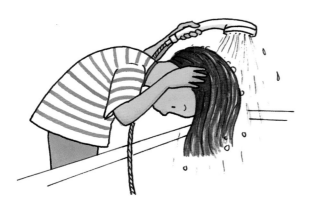

6. Dry your hair with a towel or ask an adult to dry it for you with a hairdryer.

Swimmers take care!
If you go swimming often, the chlorine in the swimming pool may damage your hair. Always use a shampoo to take the chlorine out of your hair. Use it immediately after you come out of the pool **before your hair dries.**

How you can help your hairdresser

1. Make sure you comb or brush your hair before a visit to the hairdressers.

2. Whenever you wash your hair make sure you rinse it thoroughly and dry it with a towel.

3. Try to give your hair a conditioning rinse. This gets rid of any remaining shampoo and makes it easier for you to comb through afterwards.

4. To help get knots and tangles out of your hair, start brushing from near the ends.
Brush downwards, then start a section a little higher up and brush downwards again.
Do this all the way up to the roots.

5. Never go to the hairdresser if you have head lice.

Facts about hairdressers

There are different levels of hairdressers:

Trainees. These are salon juniors who shampoo, condition and dry hair. They help with the perming and colour process and salon reception duties.

Junior hairdresser. They shampoo and condition hair but also dry the hair into shape and create a finished look. They cut, perm and colour hair.

Senior stylist or supervisor (qualified hairdresser). Their job involves different cutting techniques, perming, colouring and making sure that the clients are happy. They also help to deal with the running of the salon.

Paul, the hairdresser in this book is a senior stylist and salon owner. He employs stylists and salon juniors (trainees). During one day in his salon there are about fourteen hair-cuts as well as colourings and perms. Paul also works with a beauty therapist who does manicure, pedicure and massage.

Index

© 1998 Franklin Watts

Franklin Watts
96 Leonard Street
London
EC2A 4RH

Franklin Watts Australia
14 Mars Road
Lane Cove
NSW 2066

ISBN: 0 7496 2971 1

Dewey Decimal Classification
Number: 646.7

10 9 8 7 6 5 4 3 2 1

A CIP catalogue record for
this book is available from the
British Library.

Printed in Malaysia

Editor: Samantha Armstrong
Designer: Kirstie Billingham
Photographer: Steve Shott
Illustrations: Kim Woolley

With thanks to: Annabel, Emily
and Charlie McMahon, Matthew
Deary, Nicola and Hannah Renton,
Craig Vermay, Paul Griffin and all
the staff of Cascade Hair Salon,
Thames Road, Chiswick.

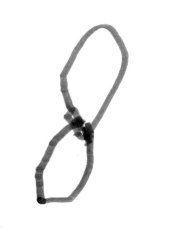